This book belongs to

Emma Harry
NGATOM

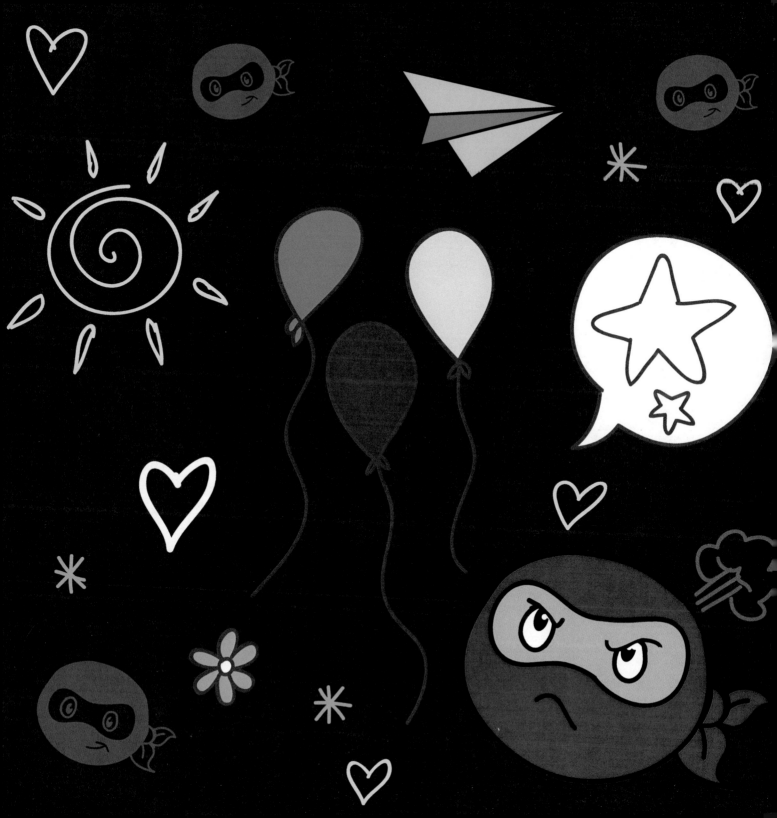

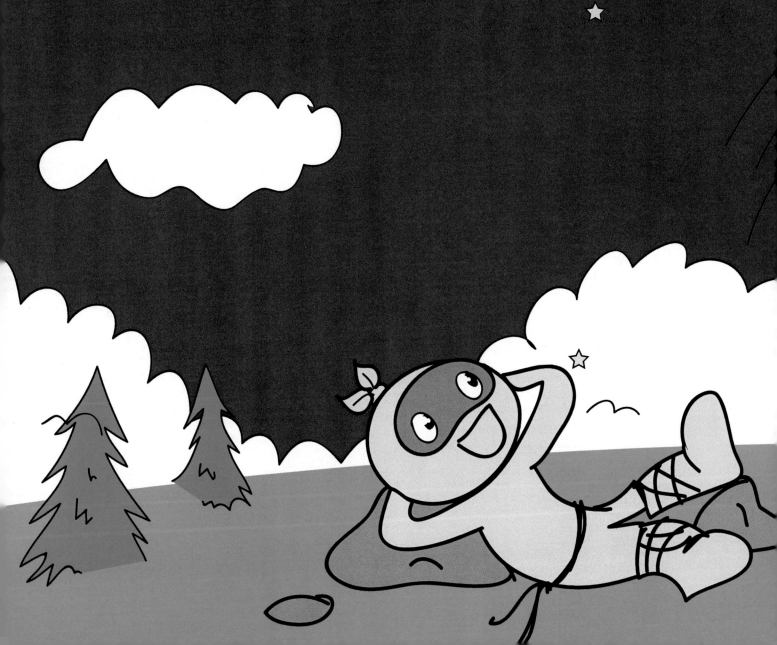

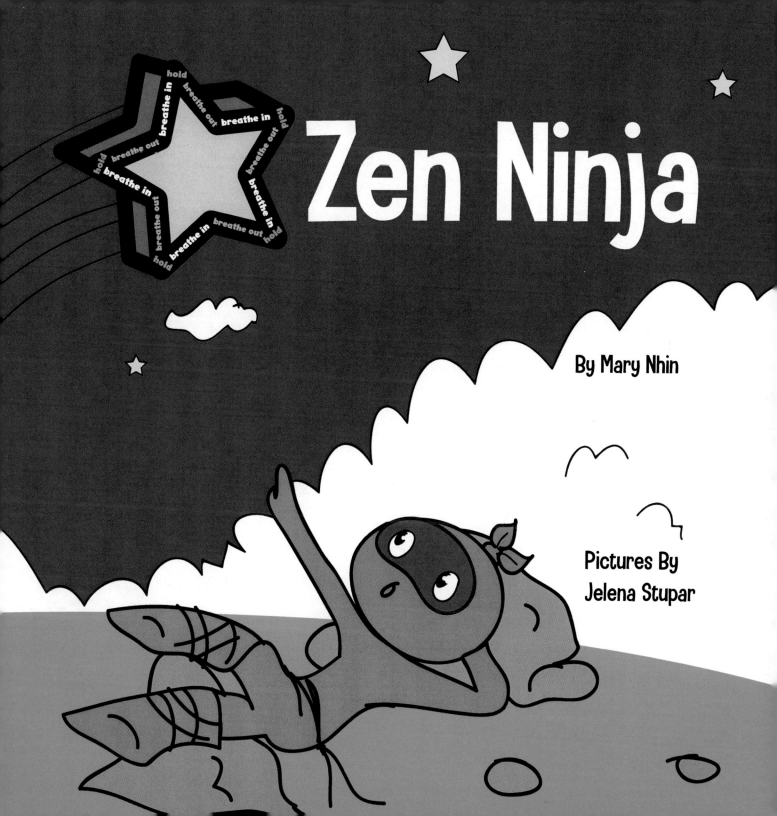

Zen Ninja

By Mary Nhin

Pictures By
Jelena Stupar

You would think that a place where kangaroos hop around and koalas sing from the trees would be a chaotic place, but it's here that Zen Ninja finds the most peace.

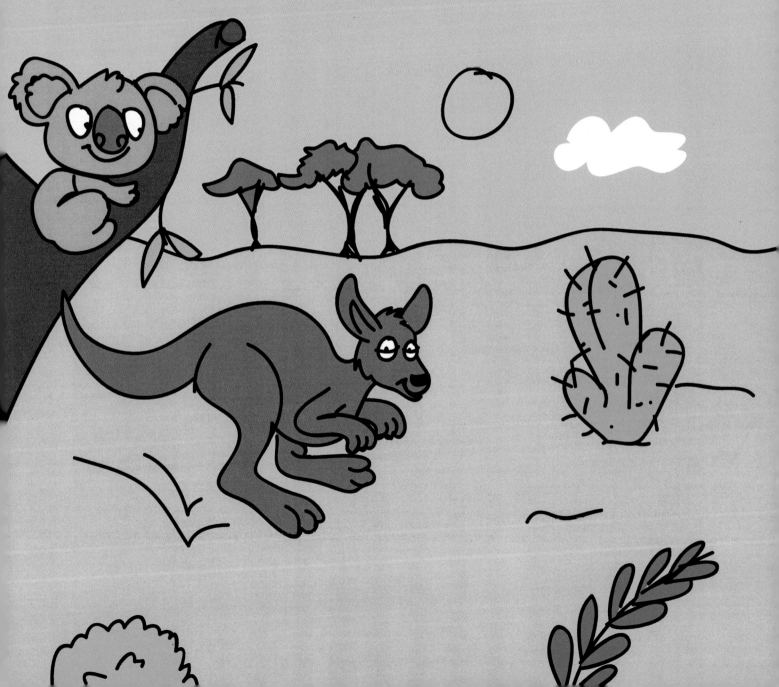

No matter what happens, the Zen Ninja takes a breath and lives by the Australian motto of "No worries".

But how does Zen Ninja stay in the zone?

Easy....

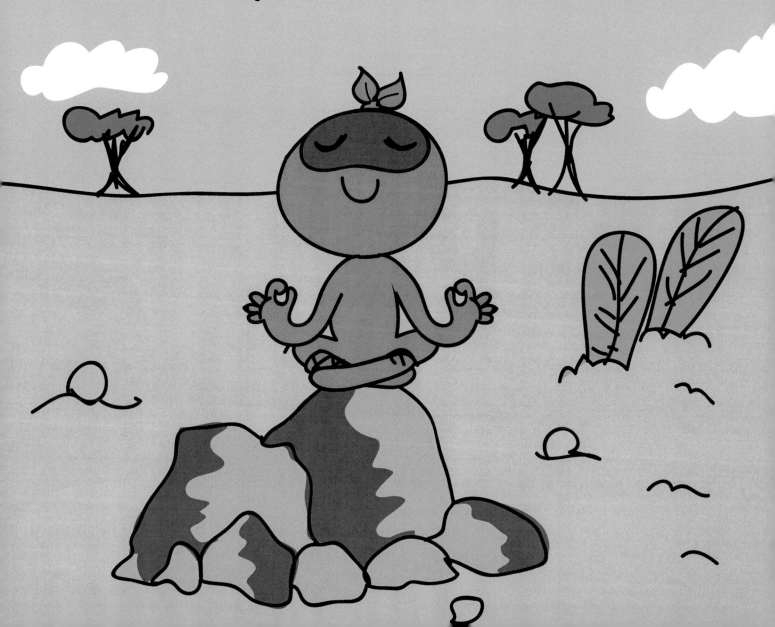

It's the Zen Ninja's 5 Star Breathing!
Each point gives you the key to calmness.
Breathe in....hold...breathe out.

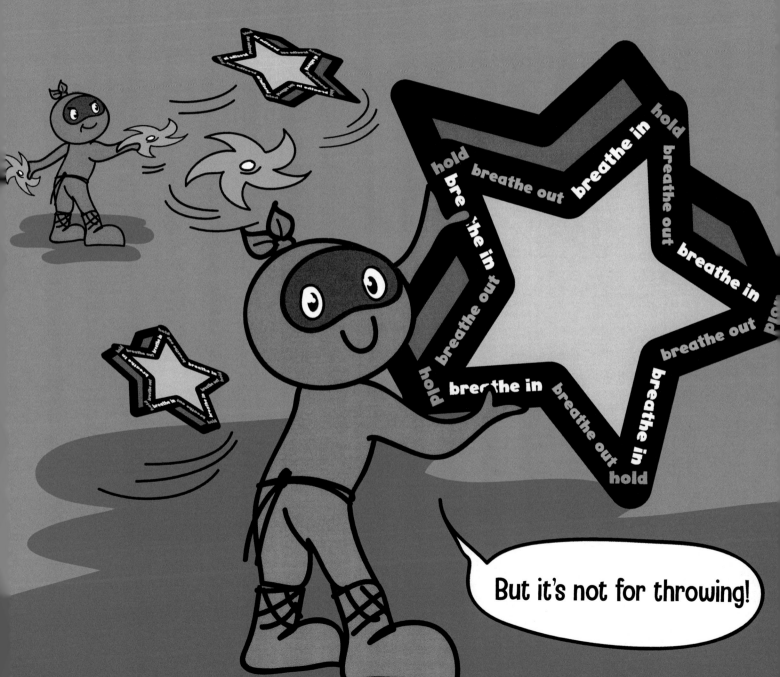

But it's not for throwing!

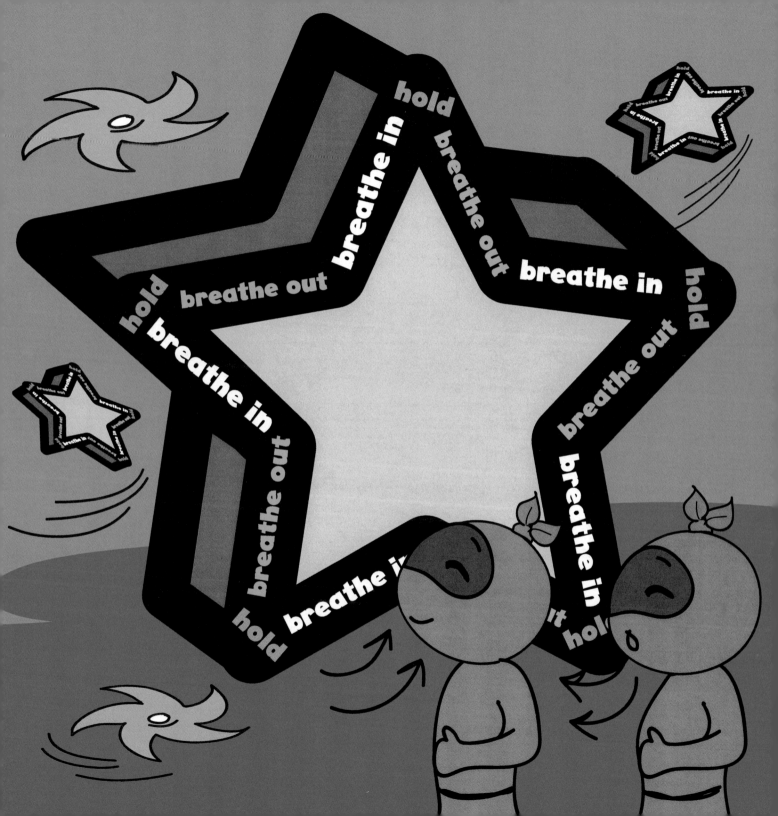

If you find yourself upset because you can't figure something out, you can calm yourself with the Zen Ninja's 5 Star!

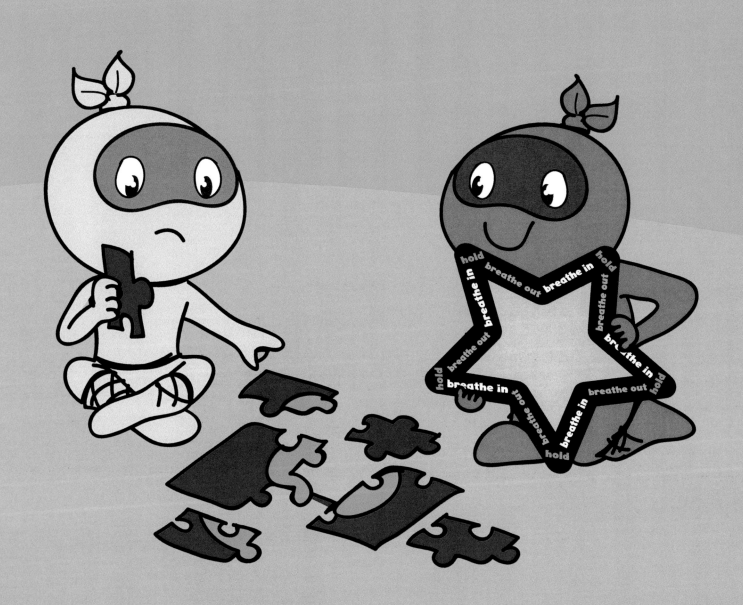

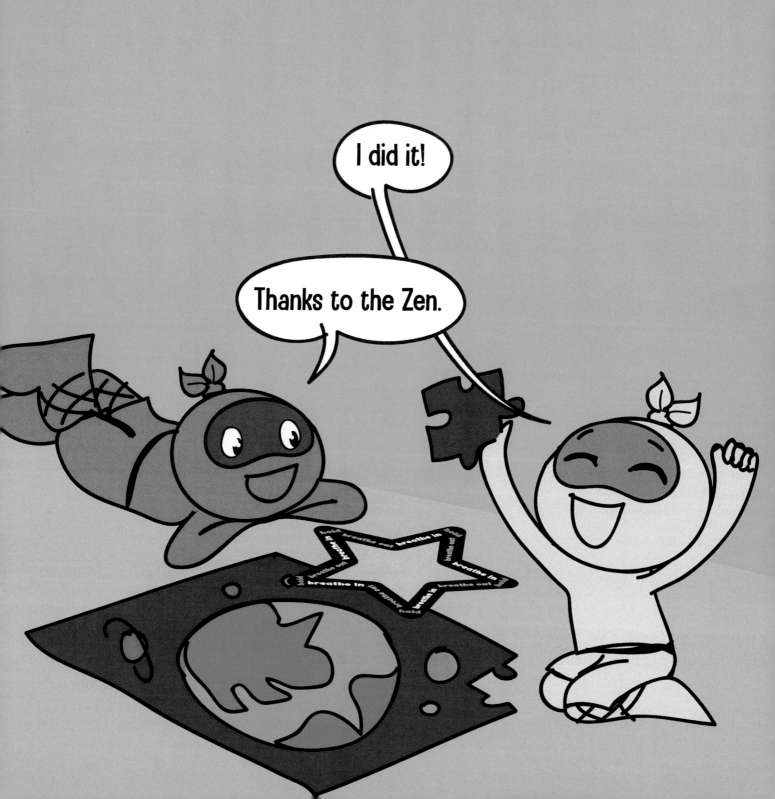

If something happens that makes you want to scream and shout...

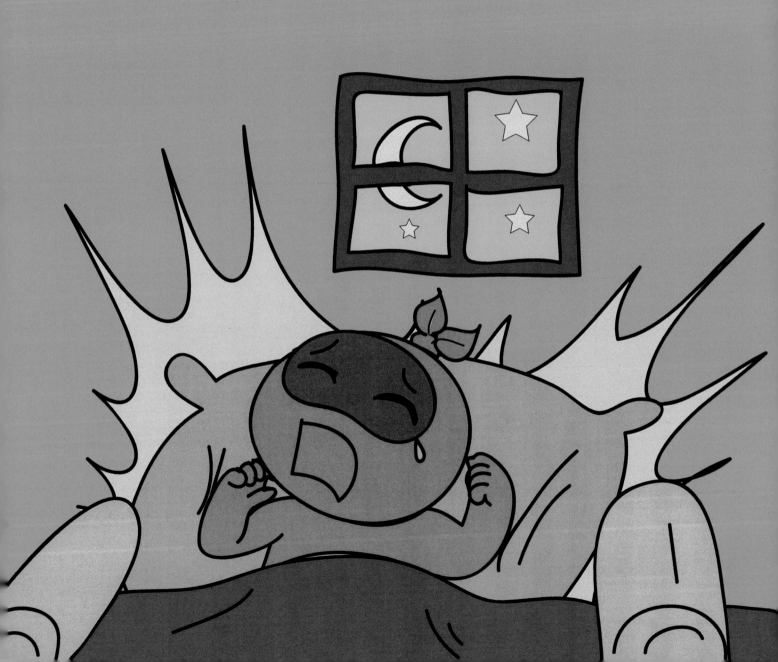

Zen Ninja's 5 Star Breathing can bring calm back to your world and help you see things differently.

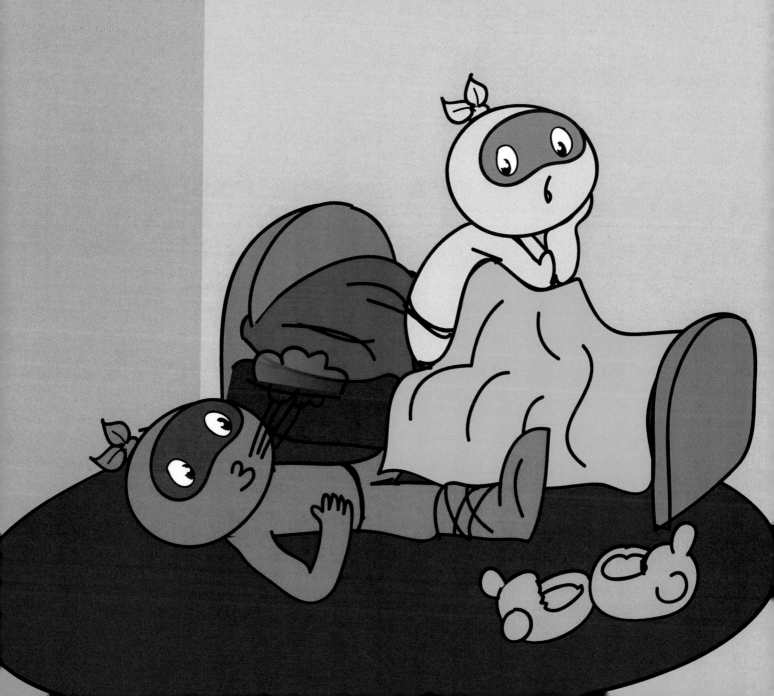

It's really easy to become Zen and calm if you follow the star.
Try it now and see how different you'll feel.

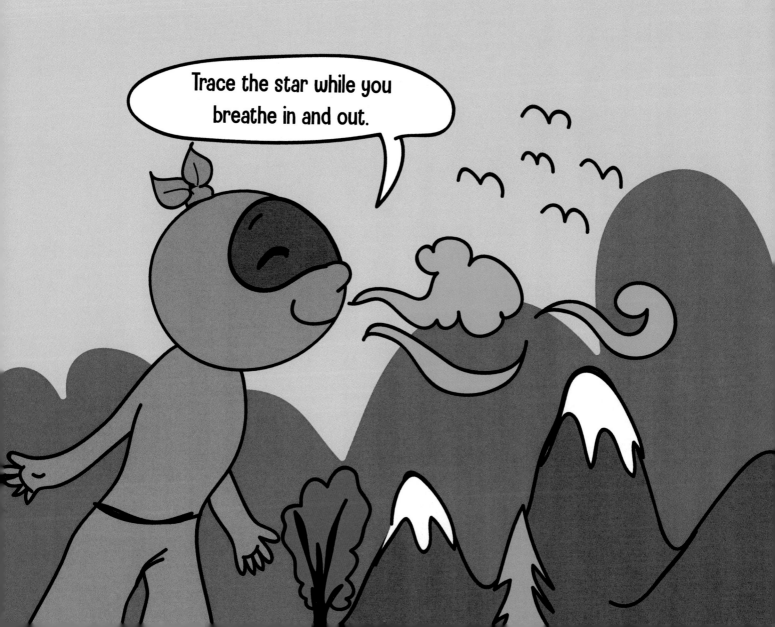

Breathe in...Hold...Breathe out.
Breathe in...Hold...Breathe out.
Breathe in...Hold...Breathe out.
Breathe in...Hold...Breathe out.
Breathe in...Hold...Breathe out.

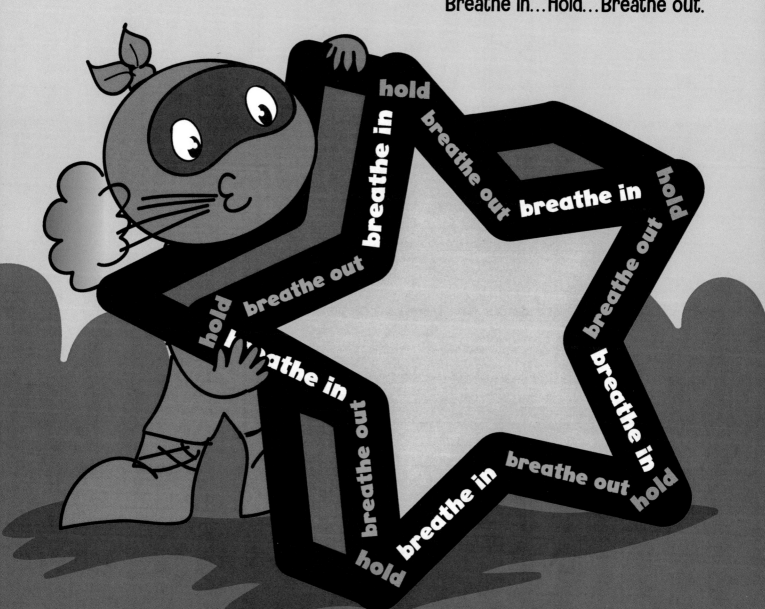

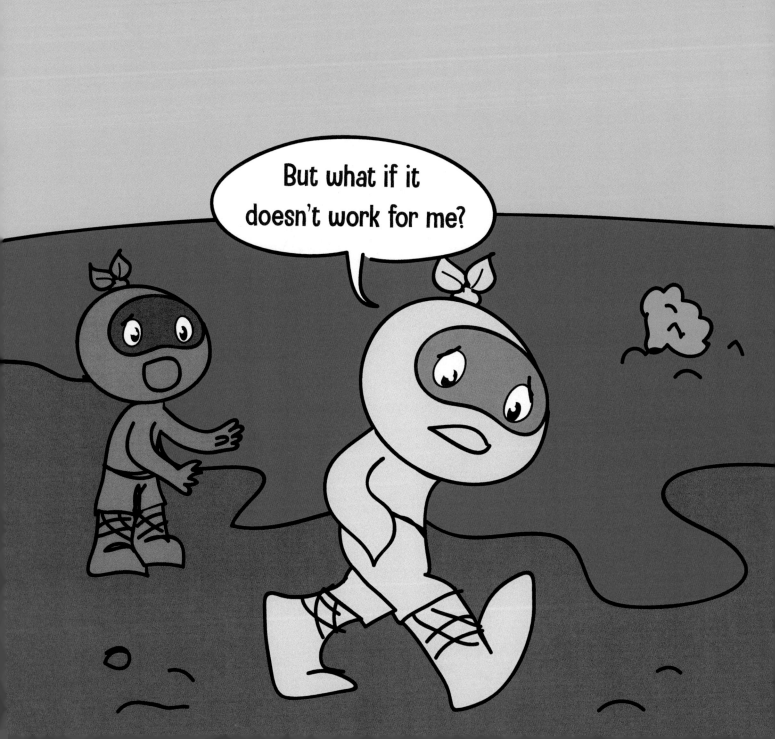

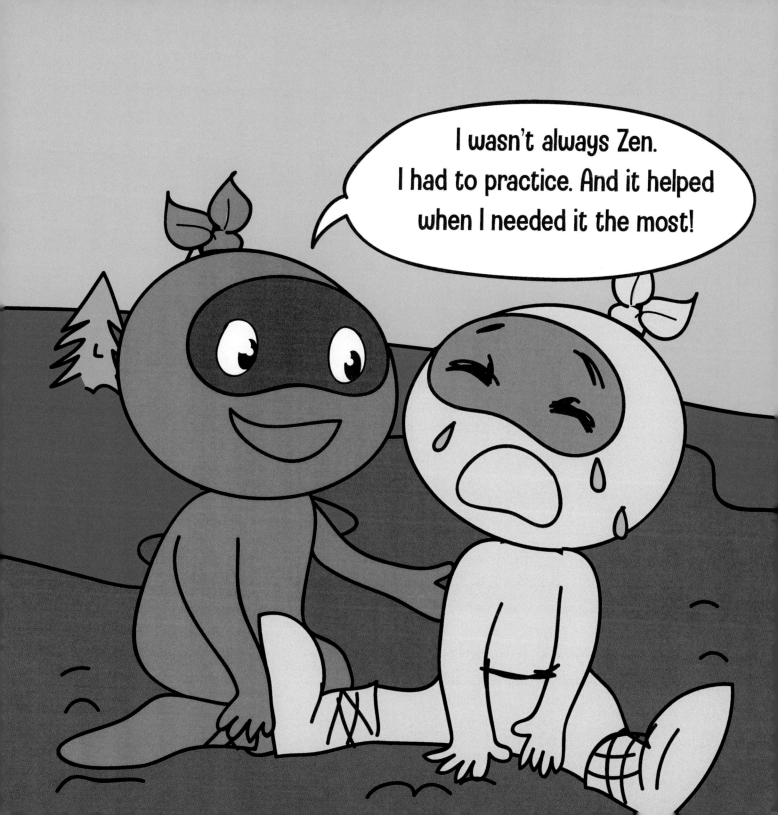

One day, Zen Ninja's parents told him that they were moving. He was going to have to leave his school and his friends. The worst part was he was going to have to start over someplace new.

This made Zen Ninja very upset and he felt really sad.

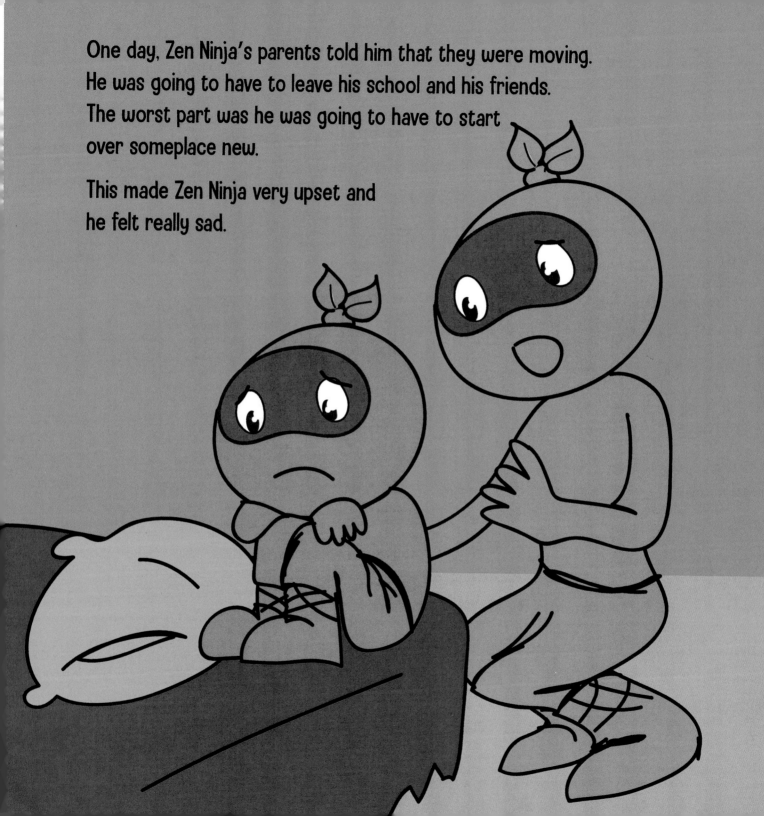

He was also very scared.

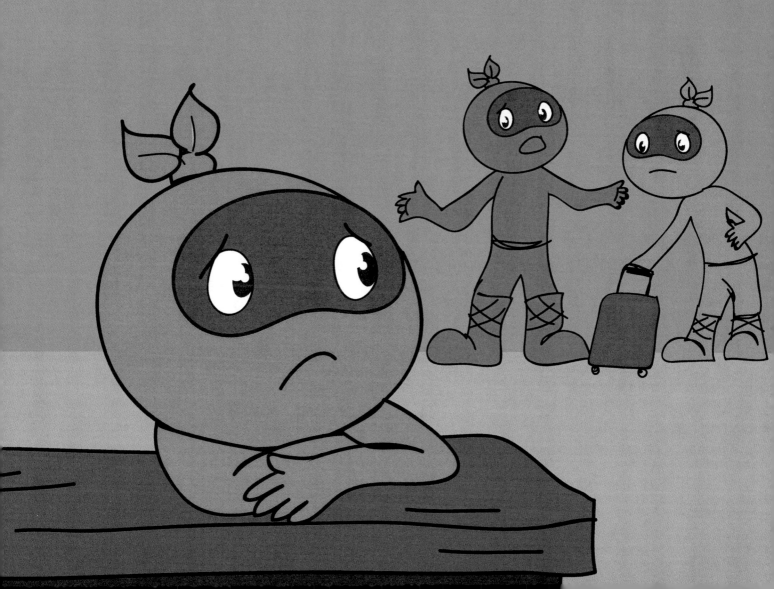

Zen Ninja's parents taught him about 5 Star Breathing. They left him to think about it.

He didn't think that it would help at first, but he tried it anyways.

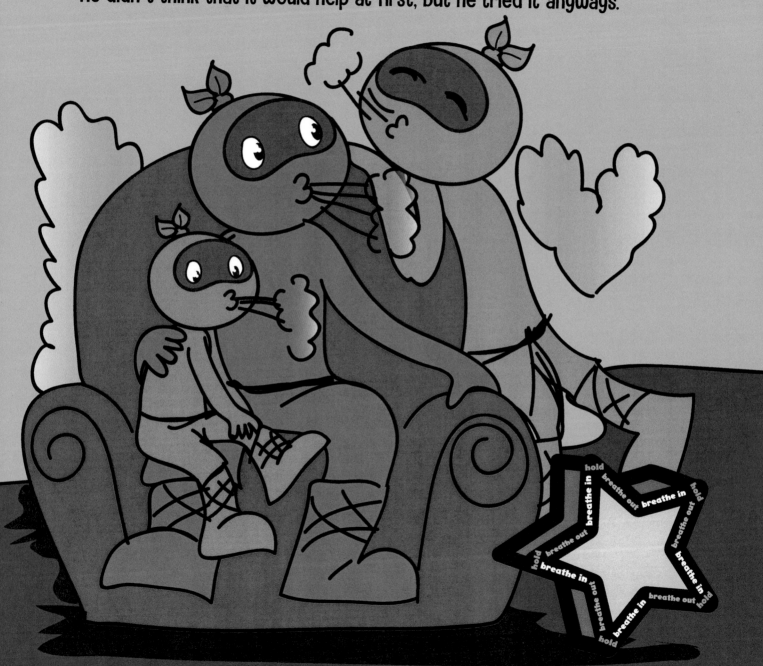

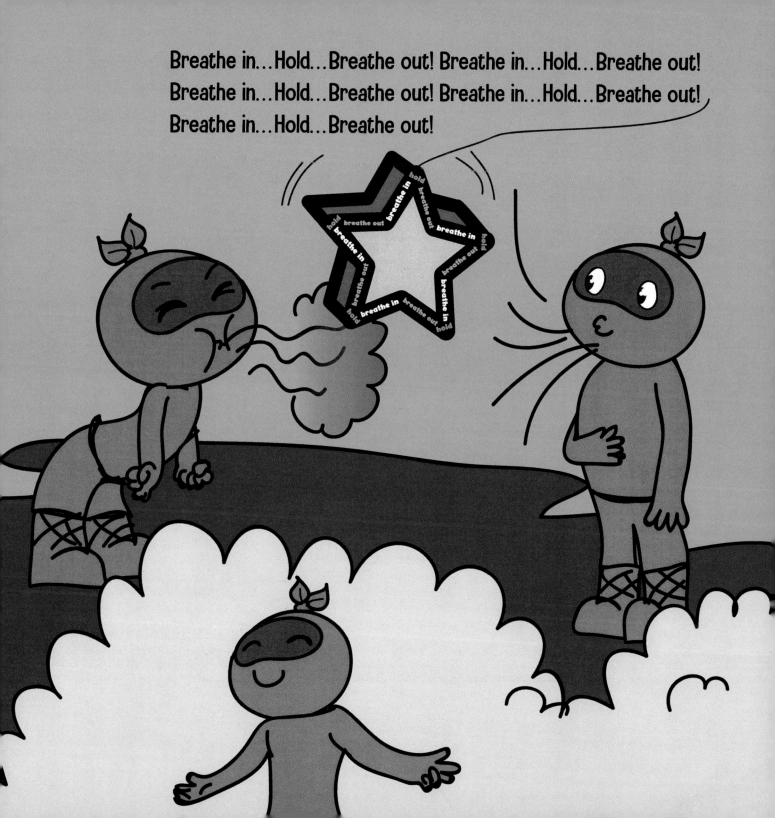

Indeed, this did make him feel better.

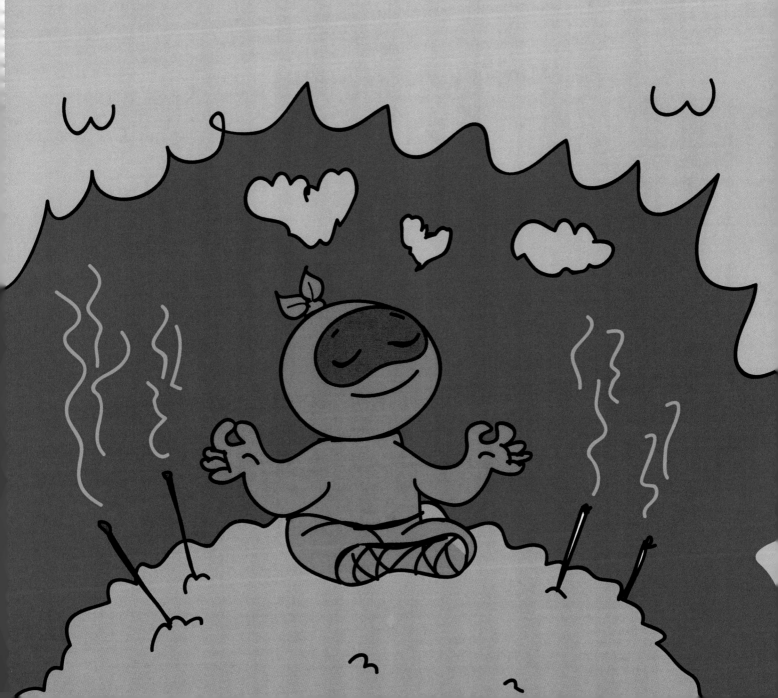

He still felt sad that he would miss his friends and his room but knew that there were more friends to be made and adventures to explore in the new neighborhood.

And with that new mindset and calm, he exclaimed...

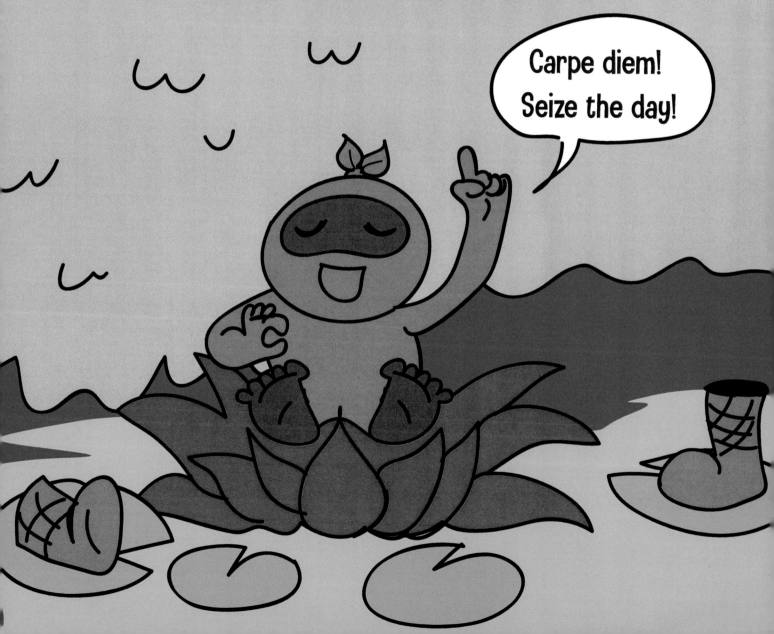

Thank you Zen Ninja for teaching me this amazing trick! Now, whenever I'm angry, stressed, or worried, I'll calm myself with your 5 Star Breathing and be Zen like you!

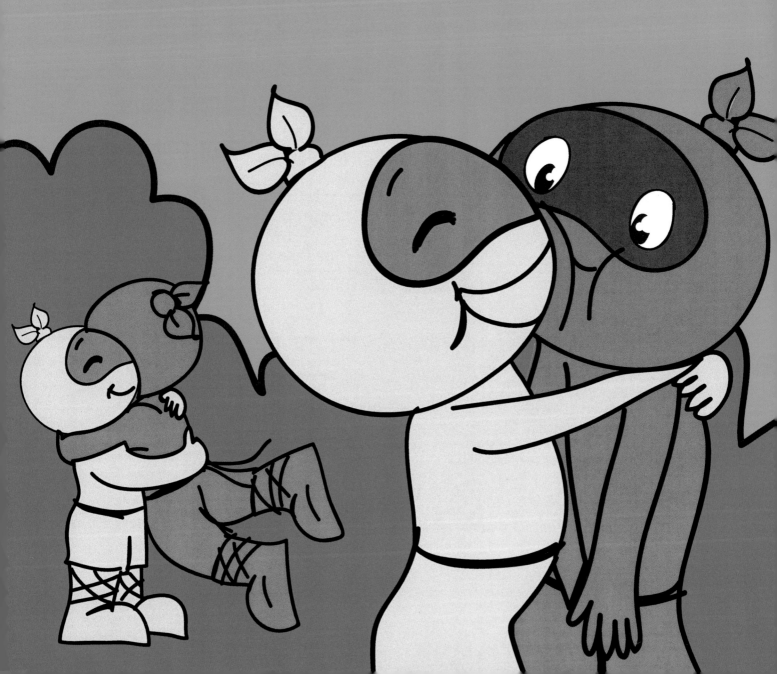

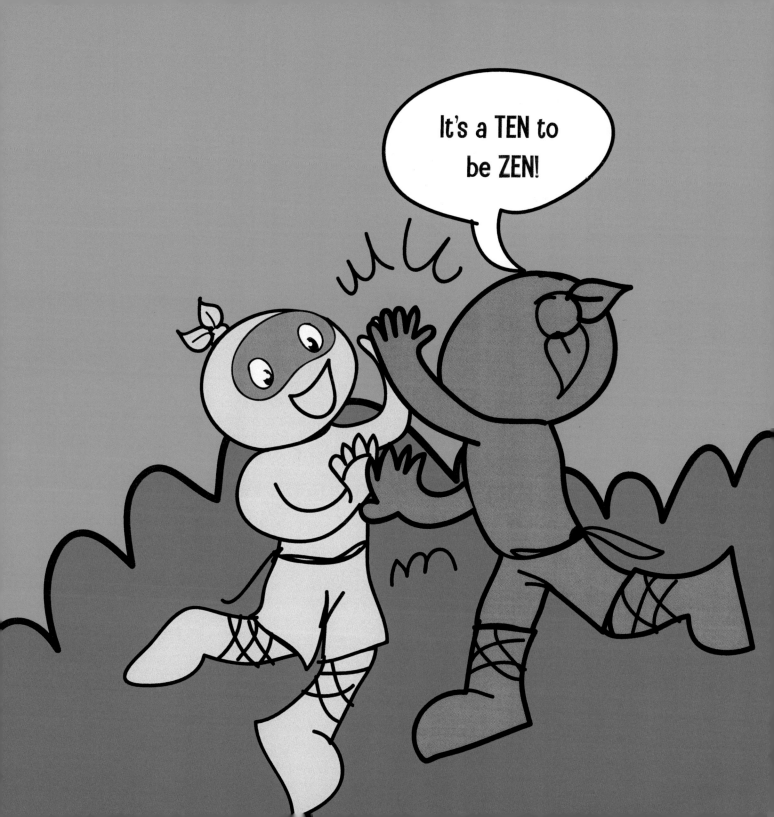

It doesn't matter if you're the new kid, a koala, or a roo...

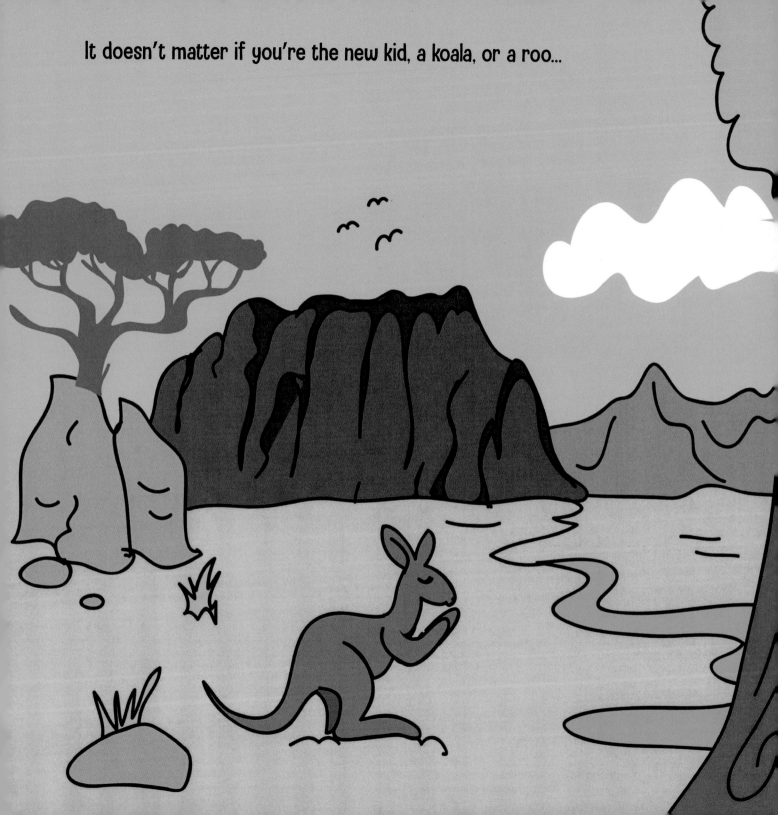

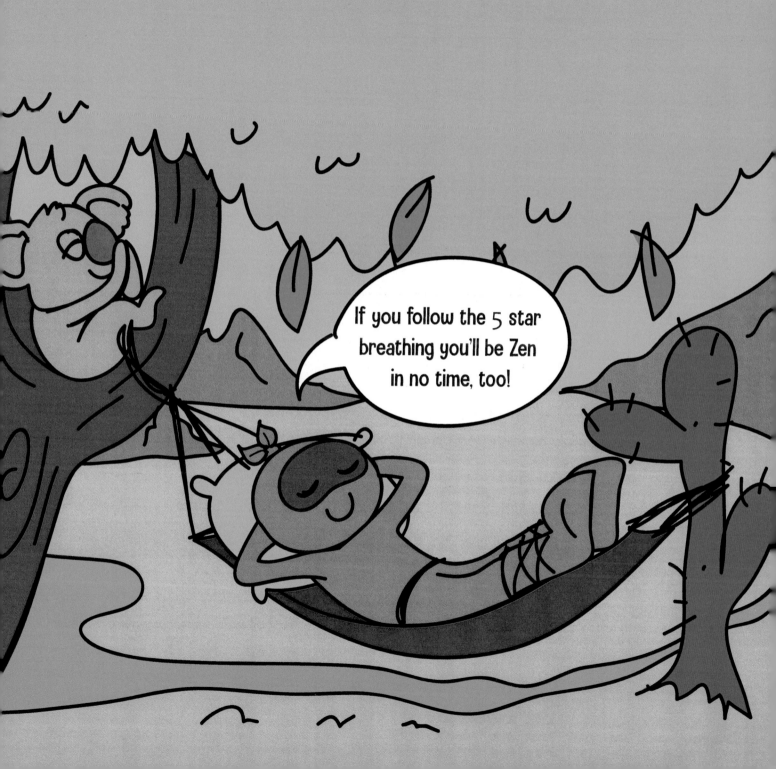

Remembering the Zen 5 Star Breathing could be your secret weapon when worry and stress begin to fill your mind.

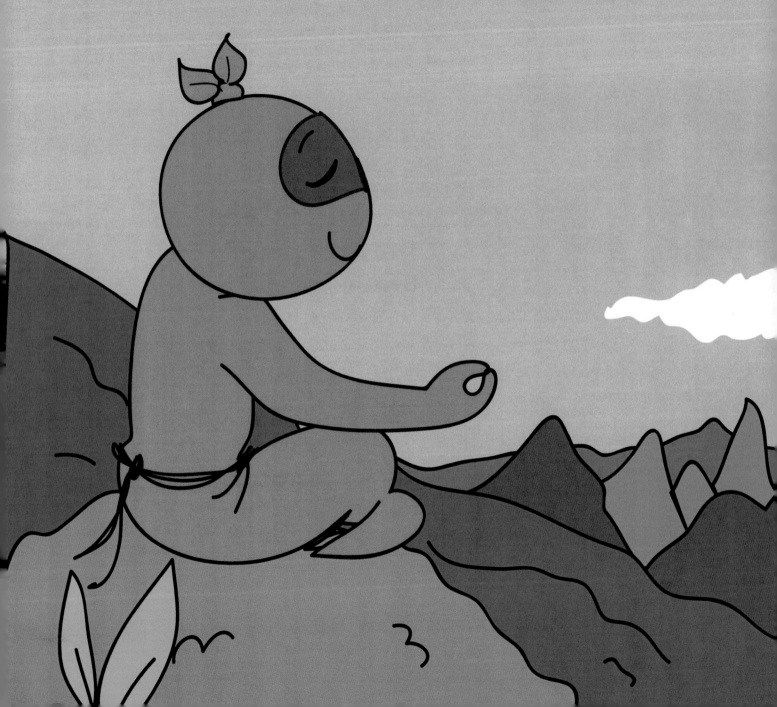

Please visit us at ninjalifehacks.tv for more lesson plans on finding your Zen.

@marynhin @GrowGrit
#NinjaLifeHacks

Mary Nhin   Grow Grit

Grow Grit

Made in the USA
Las Vegas, NV
18 May 2021